THE BALANCING ACT

Learning how to balance motherhood with fitness and nutrition

Shantel McCoy

The first step to making progress, is acknowledging the need for change. Only then will you reach your full potential.

—SHANTEL

This book is dedicated to the women. Whether you are balancing a job, parenting or anything else you may be going through in life. Take care of yourself. Love yourself. Do what it is best for you and never give up. Anything is possible with hard work and dedication.

CONTENTS

INTRODUCTION

*Challenges are what make life interesting and
Overcoming them is what makes life meaningful
—Joshua J. Marine*

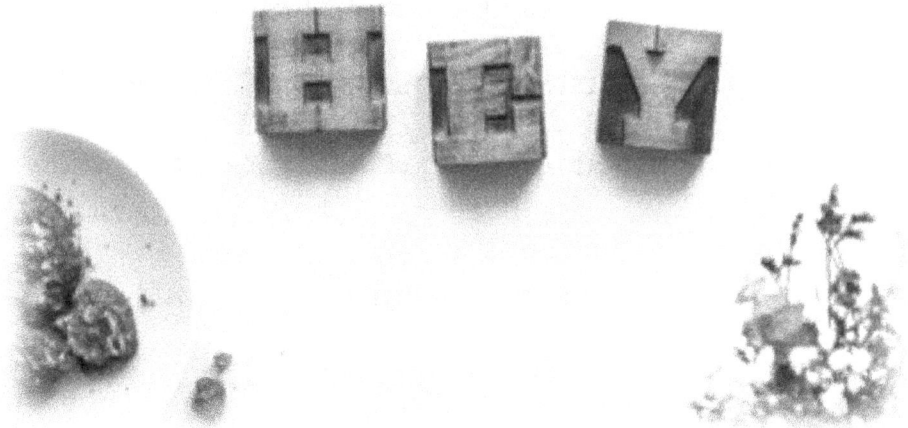

The most challenging part of being a mom is balancing parenting with self-care. We spend our days cooking, cleaning, and making sure our children's needs are met, but we forget about our own. It's hard to find time to exercise or to focus on the food we are allowing into our bodies because we put all of our energy into our children. But tell me this, if we are spending our days constantly meeting the needs of our children, how are our needs being met? I completely understand it is not easy at all. Our kids are supposed to come first. I know this may sound selfish, but actually we should be putting ourselves first. Just think of it like this, if something happened to us, who would care for our kids?

You see, I am 28 and a single mother of 5 children. I've been doing it on my own for about 7 years now. My kids are all a year or two apart in age and their ages range between 5-11 years old. As you can imagine, my hands are completely full. When I do get a break, exercise and eating healthy are usually the last things on my mind. I would go out and enjoy fast food without five little voices begging me for fries. I would walk around my house without any clothes on and a huge glass of wine and a shot of vodka. Sometimes I would skip the wine and just have vodka. I would pull all of the snacks out of the pantry and just lie in my bed and enjoy. Never once did I stop and think about the damage I was doing to my body.

Being a single mother comes with a lot of stress. It's just you. You are the only one responsible for the care of your kids. You become provider, chef, doctor, teacher and whatever else they need you to be. You stress about whether or not you are doing a good job or if you made the right decisions. You stress about bills and just being able to provide in general. Everyone have their different ways of coping with stress. Food was my coping mechanism. To an extent it still is. I could eat whole breakfast meal and still feel like needed something more. I would have snacks hidden in my room just so that they were handy when I needed them. I could sit for hours and just constantly eat and snack on cookies or chocolate. I was a stress eater and did not care. It made me feel good in that moment.

After I had my youngest daughter, I put on a few extra pounds. I didn't think too much of it because gaining weight is a normal thing when having children. But instead of trying to work it off, I got comfortable. I didn't make any attempts to exercise and my diet consisted of pancakes with extra syrup for breakfast, four wings and fries for lunch and a juicy cheeseburger and fries for dinner. I didn't drink water so the next best thing was tea with extra sugar or soda. I hated water so much that if I really had to drink it, I would add sugar to it. Some days I would drink energy drinks just to make it through the day. This was something that went on for years, but I guess it had finally started to catch up with me. Before I knew it, I was hitting 160lbs. For someone that is only 4ft and 11in tall, it was not a good look. I refuse to walk around looking like an Umpa Lumpa. I remember my last doctor's visit; he told me that if I put on any more weight, I would be hitting obesity. Once I realized that my weight was continuously going up and I couldn't fit into my jeans anymore, I knew I needed to make some changes.

Not only was I putting on more weight, but I was beginning to experience physical pain as well. I would get terrible back pains and migraines. I mean it got bad to the point where I would cry like a baby. I would go back and forth to the ER, but they could not determine the cause of the pain. They would just give me medicine and send me home. At one point it got so bad that it would wake me up out of my sleep and I was unable to move. I knew at that point that something was really wrong.

I decided to go to a different hospital. I told them about all of the symptoms I was having. They asked me questions like, what was I doing right before the pain started? How often do I move around? What type of foods do I eat? My answers were, I had either just finished eating or had drank a soda, I get up to feed my kids and clean a little but other than that I am in my bed, and you don't even want to know the kind of food I eat. The look on that Doctor's face was priceless. He looked at me as if to say, "Well duhhhh." But instead he politely said, "I have an idea of what the problem could be but I am going to run some test to be sure." He then explained to me that it could possibly be my gallbladder. Although there are a number of reasons why people have issues with their gallbladder, a poor diet can be one of them. Once it was confirmed that my gallbladder was inflamed, he said that the only option would be surgery to remove it.

You would think after having five C-sections, I wouldn't be the least bit worried. But I was terrified. It made me take a deeper look at my life. How could I possibly care for 5 little people and I can't take care of myself? What would happen to them if something happened to me? I needed to make some changes. I needed to make sure that I could take care of them and not hand them the responsibility of having to take care of me. I needed to start taking care of me.

The surgery was a success. Once I was fully recovered, I didn't feel any more of that pain. That was a huge relief because I was able to try to focus on my diet and exercise. It was not easy at all to make the changes. I didn't know where to begin as far as exercising. I didn't have the energy for it. I was self-conscious. I felt so embarrassed trying to do jumping jacks or any exercise that involved standing up and moving. Every time I would try to start exercising, my kids would need something. It was always something. I would just stop and try again the next day. I did that pretty much every day.

I had no clue where to begin with eating healthy. My body was hooked on sweets. I craved burgers and pizza. I did not want to trade my juicy burgers for some leaves. Like seriously, what is life without burgers and pizza? But I had to suck it up and figure it out if I wanted to have any chance at living longer and dropping this weight. I am all that my kids have. I knew that this was going to be a long and hard process. But it had to be done.

Do you want to know what I did to change my lifestyle while taking care of 5 kids on my own? Don't worry; I won't keep it a secret. I wish someone would've told me to be honest. If you keep reading, all of my secrets are here in this book. Hopefully you find them helpful also.

As an added bonus, you will find helpful organizers to get you started on your fitness and nutrition journey. Also, I have included a few beginner exercise routines, meal prep ideas and my top 5 favorite YouTube channels.

AS A PARENT, YOU MUST DO THIS

*You will never change your life until you
Change something you do daily. The secret
Of your success is found in your daily routine
—John C. Maxwell*

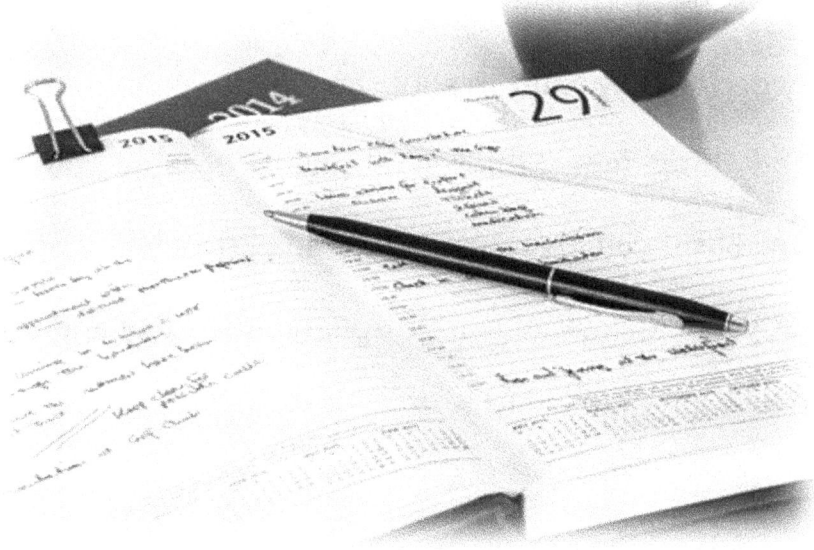

I Know. Trying to get more than one child on the same routine is like trying to get toddlers to sit still for a picture. It seems impossible. But I guarantee you, it isn't at all.

Children need a routine to help them get through their day. You need them to have a routine to get through yours. If you are just letting them wonder around and do their own thing and go to sleep when they decide they want to shut their eyes, you will never get anything done. Children ultimately do what you allow. But if you give them a schedule, they will know what your expectations are throughout the day and that will become their routine.

Being a young mother with multiple kids, a routine was a must. It wasn't a strict routine, but I had to have some kind of down time to allow myself to regroup and stay sane. By my kids being so close in age, I had to make sure I had my older kids on a sleep schedule so that I could tend to the baby without being completely exhausted. I didn't really have a routine during the day. Although, I did make sure that they took naps in the afternoon. Naps prevented them from being cranky and me from having a meltdown.

Although I kind of had a little routine down, all I could think to do is either sleep or watch TV. This is typical because you have to take time to rest when they are resting or just enjoy the quiet time. As they got older, I began to add to their routine. So, along with bedtime and naptime, I had a set time for breakfast, lunch and dinner. They also had a playtime and bath time. When they began going to school, I added chores and studying to their routine.

Some people will say that implementing a routine like that is like you are a drill sergeant and they are your cadets. That is far from the truth. Children need routine and structure. They need to have their day planned out that way they know what you are expecting from them. It also helps them out in the long run.

By having them on a routine, it teaches them time management. They will grow up knowing how to plan out their days, which will come in handy when they have to get a job. It also teaches them to be organized. You will notice once they are familiar with the routine, you won't have to go behind them as much to remind them of what they should be doing. That also teaches them to be independent and learn to do things on their own.

They are not the only ones who reap the benefits. A routine will work wonders for you. It just makes your job a little more easier. You get to have that downtime and get some stuff done. You will be able to set your own schedule within their schedule. This will be beneficial for when you start your fitness and nutrition journey. You can schedule your exercising for when they are napping or do meal prep when they go to bed.

It is not an easy task finding and sticking to a routine, but once you get the hang of it, it will begin to get easier.

I broke my routine down into three parts, morning, noon and night. Here is an example of the routine I used:

Morning

- 6am– Wake everyone up
- 6:30–7:15am– Kids get ready for school
- 7:20am– Walk kids to the bus stop
- 7:45am– Breakfast for me and my daughter
- 8am– Learning time
- 10am– TV Time
- 11am– Nap Time

Noon

- 11:30am– Exercise
- 12:15pm– 1pm– Research diet plan
- 1pm–2pm – Rest/ Quiet time
- 2:05pm– Naptime over
- 2:10pm– Lunch time
- 2:45pm– Big kids come home
- 3pm– Homework
- 3:45pm– 4:15pm– Chores
- 4:30pm– 5:15pm– Playtime/ TV
- 5:30pm– Get school stuff ready for the next day

Evening

- 6pm– Dinner
- 6:45pm– Bath time
- 7:30pm– Bedtime story
- 8pm– Bedtime
- 8:30pm–9pm– Exercise
- 9:10pm– Shower/ bedtime

This is the routine I used when my kids were in school. This routine was a little more difficult to stick with because they were used to our old routine. I had to work more with the school kids because after a long they of school they were ready to just come home and either play or sleep. But as time went on they adjusted to it.

My kids, eventually, started liking the routine. They started to watch the clock for the next task. My daughter loved learn and play time and TV time winded her down so that she could take her nap. The time frame coordinated well with bedtime. I didn't have to go through much to get them to sleep. They knew that right after story time was bedtime and they would give me a hug and kiss and went right to sleep. We had some off days but for the most part, the routine was working out.

It took me a while to create my own routine. Honestly, I didn't think about it until I had to. Even then it was still a struggle because I wasn't a very active or healthy person. I had little knowledge about exercising and eating right and that made it harder for me because I didn't know where to start. I figured exercising would be the easiest so I started there.

With their routine already in place, I already had an idea of how I could plan out my routine. During naptime, I would exercise for 30-45min. I didn't have money for fancy gym equipment or to buy the exercise DVD's. I had to improvise and find a routine that worked for me and that I didn't have to pay for. So for a period of time, I was using the exercise videos that were available through my cable provider. As far as changing the way that I ate, I put that on hold until I did a little research. So, I would just set aside my exercise time and use my other free time to research and take care of whatever else needed to be taken care of.

FINDING THE RIGHT EXERCISE ROUTINE

Giving up is not an option

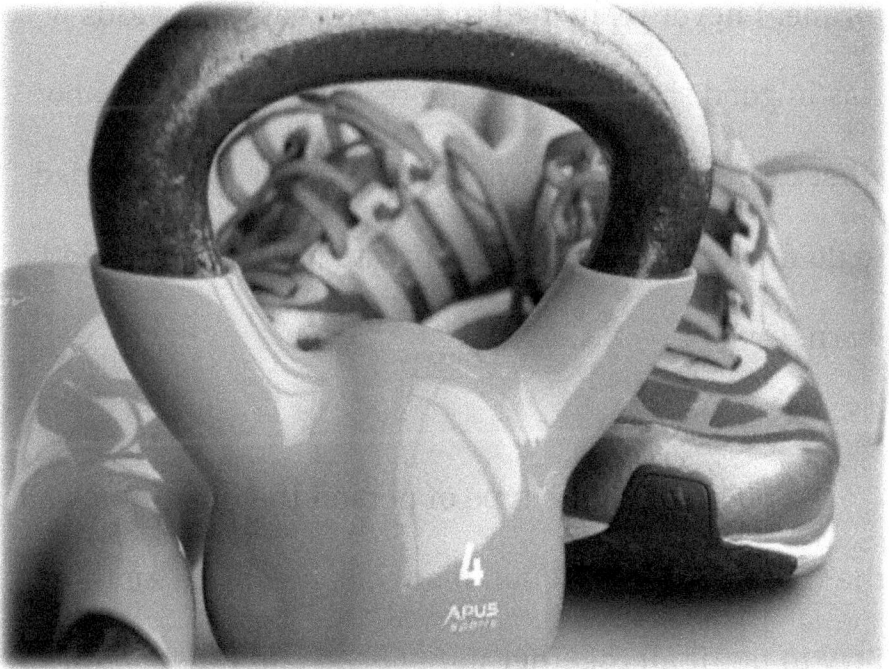

Finding the right exercise routine is not an easy task. You have to ask yourself, "What part of my body do I need to work on?" Once you have that question answered, you have to find a workout that caters to those needs.

Finding an exercise routine was the hardest part for me. I never really had to exercise before my kids. I was in good shape and had no reason to. I didn't know what exercise to do for what body part or that I needed to do my legs and arms on separate days. But boy did I learn.

You see, I'm the type of person that just jumps all the way in. No instruction manuals, no advice, nothing. I try to put it all together in my head and I just go for it.

But this right here taught me a valuable lesson, Research.

After a few days of doing it my way, my entire body was sore. I almost wanted to give up. I could barely move my arms and legs and my abdomen was on fire. I was doing way too much, way too soon. I decided to take a break and do some research. It's amazing how much information you can find out online and how many videos are posted telling you exactly what you need to know. The videos I watched through my cable provider were just teaching different exercises. They weren't telling me the proper way to use those exercises. That's why I was in so much pain. I was doing the exercises, but I was doing them all wrong.

In my search I came across some workout challenges/routines. I literally typed, exercise routine for beginners in the google search bar and a ton of websites popped up. I took the shortcut and clicked on images. They have workouts on there to fit anybody's routine. I mean hundreds of workouts. It was so many that it took me a while to figure out which one would work for me. So, I ended up choosing two.

I decided to go with a 30 day squat challenge and a 24 day ab workout. The good thing about the challenge is that they both started off easy and had you work your way up to longer and harder exercises. (See the back of the book for the exact challenges I used). I couldn't wait for my body to heal so I could start my challenge.

Another site I found very helpful was YouTube. YouTube and I became best friend. It was like a broke person's guide to fitness. They had videos for everything. They showed what exercises worked for what part of the body. They gave in detail how to schedule your exercise routine. They even had dance workout videos. So, you mean to tell me I can dance and exercise at the same time? If I wasn't motivated before, I was definitely motivated now. I love dancing, so being able to dance and get in shape at the same time was music to my ears. Now I had to map it out.

I decided I would stick to the challenges. Kind of like a 30 day warm up. That would allow my body to adjust to exercising regularly and loosen up my muscles. It would also help me to better my day to day workout routine. I wanted to be ready for my YouTube workout. I had already started putting together a playlist of the different exercises I would try.

About halfway through the challenges, I became anxious about starting my YouTube workout. So I decided to do the challenges during naptime and do 15min of the YouTube workout before bed. I wanted to do more, but I didn't want to put too much on me like before. I felt so accomplished. I was actually exercising regularly. After a few weeks, I started noticing results. My baby weight was slowly but surely dropping off.

Just by doing some research and learning how to better organize my day, I was finally able to exercise on a regular basis. It is important to remember, when coming up with your exercise routines, to take breaks. Take like 2 or 3 days out of the week and just allow your body to rest. You can also schedule your workouts every other day and work your way up to exercising on a day to day basis. Whatever works best for you. Just remember to rest and stay hydrated in between workouts.

WHAT TO DO WHEN YOUR KIDS ARE HOME FOR THE SUMMER?

It always seem impossible, until it is done
–Nelson Mandela

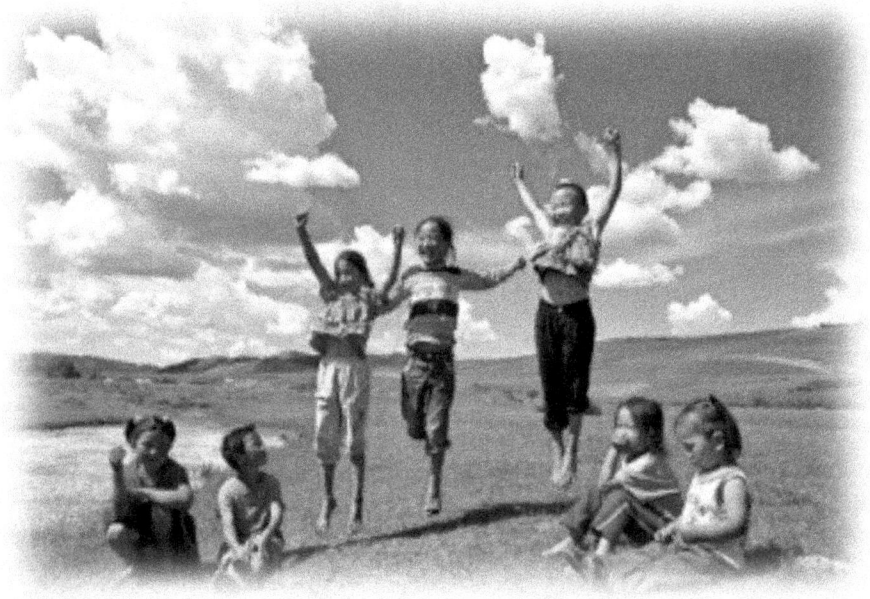

So, summertime is here and school is out. You already have your routine on track, but now you have to find a way to switch it up to accommodate your kids without completely messing up your workout schedule. How is that even possible?

It's kind of simple. Just include them. You may have to make a few adjustments and allow them time to get the hang of it, but it is absolutely doable.

As your kids get older, naptime sort of fades away. This means that you will now have to find something to substitute naptime. At the beginning of your workout, allow them to join in. Let's face it, they are going to be right there watching and bugging you anyway. You might as well put them to work. By doing this, not only are you able to still workout, but you are showing your kids how to incorporate exercise in their day. Not to mention, this could be perfect for bonding time. Kids don't care what you all are doing, as long as they have your attention and are interacting with you. I guarantee they will love it.

Another thing I started doing is going outside with them during my exercise time. I would play catch with them or play tag, you're it. It's good to switch things up when you have children. Kids get bored and need different activities to keep their attention. So, by me taking them outside during my time, they came up with ways to incorporate my exercises into whatever we were doing outside.

Say for instance, when we played tag, instead of the person freezing once they are tagged, they changed

it to having the person run in place. They would
randomly stop playing and do some of the warm up
exercises. At times, we would just do the whole workout
routine and they each took turns being the instructor.
Let me tell you, letting a child feel like they are in
charge for a little while, does wonders for their self-
esteem and helps build their confidence. My kids loved
it. They looked forward to it. All of this fun we were
having and still managed to exercise in the process.

When including the children, try to make your in-
home workout as fun as possible. Include your children
in some of the decision making. That way they would
stay motivated to do it and you won't have to worry
about constant interruptions. I used to find kid friendly
exercises on YouTube and made it like it was their
exercise time. Or I would put on a dance workout and

make it like we were learning new dance moves. Once they started getting into the routine, I allowed them to take turns picking out which workout we would do and what songs we would listen to during our workout. This gave them something to look forward to. Therefore, they were ready and willing to participate in exercise time.

Every day didn't go as smooth as it sounds. There were days where one of my kids felt like they wanted to pick with the others. Sometimes, they just wanted to lie around the house. Other times, there would be no cooperation from anyone. Some days were filled with punishments and time outs. While other days, I just gave up.

Do not go into this thinking it's going to be easy because it's not. Kids require constant attention and have constant needs. That is why a good routine is beneficial to you all. That way they already know what to expect throughout the day. So, even if you all are having a bad day, try to stick to the routine as much as you can. That way they know that no matter what kind of day they are having, dinner will still be at 6pm and they will be in bed by 8pm. It takes a while, but it gets easier over time.

THE STRUGGLES OF HEALTHY EATING

*Discipline is the bridge between goals
And accomplishments
— Jim Rohn*

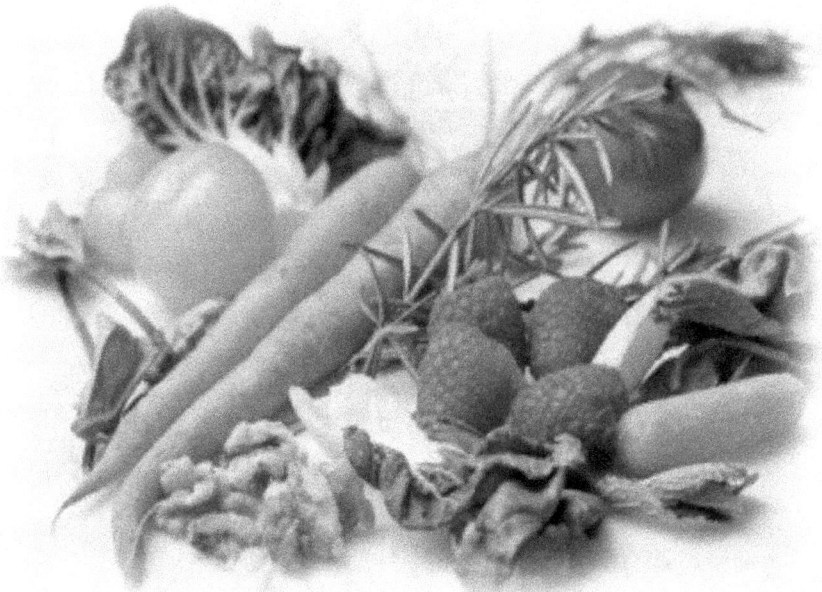

Here comes the hard part, changing my diet. When I tell you it was hard, IT WAS HARD! Not to mention, I was a picky eater and vegetables were never on my menu. I didn't know how I was going to do this. How could I give up everything I loved to eat for everything I hated?

My cabinets were stuffed with all kinds of sweets; cakes, cookies and chocolate. You name it, I'm sure I had it. I had all kinds of meat in my freezer, like burgers, steaks, pork chops, ground beef and hot dogs. My refrigerator was filled with juice, soda and tea. I had nothing healthy in sight.

Of course, my first order of business was to get rid of all of the unhealthy food, which was just about everything. It took me a while to get it done. You are crazy if you thought I was just going to throw it away. I did what any normal person would do. I waited until we ate all of the food we had in the house, to start my nutritional journey. Two things I didn't waste were food and money. Healthy had to wait. I know that was a bad decision on my part, but I wanted to enjoy it before it was gone. I told myself that I was going to be serious about it. Which meant the next time I went to the store, I would not be bringing home any of that food.

While I was taking the time to get rid of the unhealthy food, I started my grocery list. Yes, I cheated. I needed some cookies and burgers to reward myself for doing well. Don't laugh, it was a process. I didn't have it in me to go all in. I didn't know how to go all in. I couldn't resist the food that I practically grew up on.

I had to conduct numerous interviews with people that I knew ate healthy. I was lost. I didn't know where to begin. I did surveys to see what foods were recommended the most. I asked around for the best but cheapest place to shop for healthy foods. I researched meals that I could possibly make to substitute my craving for burgers. This was some work.

After doing my research, I realized that eating healthy would take up a lot of time and money. So, I decided to take baby steps. I knew I could tolerate fruit, so I started with that. I also started cutting back on the amount of unhealthy food I ate. So, instead of completely filling my plate up, I cut my serving size in half. Cutting out sodas wasn't as hard as I thought it would be. Once I stopped buying them, I stopped drinking them and didn't really get an urge to have them anymore. I still drank tea, but found a brand that didn't contain as much sugar. I started buying more water than I did juice. That way when I got thirsty, I would have to either drink water to make my juice last, or water would be all that I had left after my juice was gone. Of course, I had to make my juice last. I couldn't go a day without it. My strategies became very helpful in the process. By me cutting back on the unhealthy foods, I started slowly eliminating them all together.

Another important thing, when considering eating healthy, is that everyone else around you eats healthy also. It's a hard task to finish your fruit and veggies when people around you are eating steaks and cakes. This felt like this was going to be theee most challenging part of the process. Try telling a child that their bellies will no longer be filled with sugars and sweets and they have to cut back on juice. Well now, try telling 5. I was having a hard enough time adjusting to this new way of eating, so I knew my kids were not going to like it at all. I felt like getting them to exercise was a piece of cake compared to what I was about to have them do. But I had to do what I had to do.

I started using Pinterest for creative and budget friendly ideas to ease children into healthy eating. Pinterest became a go to site for pretty much everything involving healthy eating. They have so much information and ideas that you can't really come up with a good enough excuse as to why you are not doing it. I was able to find fun recipes and snack ideas to help my kids along the process. I found ideas about the kind of conversations I could have with them to get them to give it a try. I found things for me to read to me to give it a try. I knew this was going to be a long and hard process, but I had to start somewhere.

As I said before, I started with fruit. So, I also started my kids with fruit. I would eat an apple for breakfast with my cereal and would add bananas, strawberries or blueberries to their oatmeal. Sometimes for lunch, I would let them pick one fruit a piece, and let them make a fruit salad. That idea was a hit. They started asking for fruits more and more often. I would often let them have a fruit and veggie party. They loved that idea. They were able to pick out the fruits and veggies and pick either a movie or some music and have a party while they were eating healthy. Now that I had worked the fruits in, it was on to the hard stuff, veggies.

I hate vegetables. There is no other way to say it. There is no sugar coating. I hate them. I always have for as long as I can remember. Although I hated them, I would still give them to my kids when I cooked dinner. So, this process would be much harder for me then it would be for them. I couldn't stand the thought of chewing on some leaves. I couldn't stand the way they smelled. I just wasn't having it. I honestly did not know how I was going to do this. Even Pinterest motivational blogs and quotes didn't work. So, I just worked on getting my kids to eat them more. My kids knew that I wanted to be healthier, so they often made me put veggies on my plate. That's all I did was put them on my plate. When they weren't looking, I threw them right in the trash. I sound like a kid, I know. I just couldn't bring myself to do it. I felt like this was a failed mission.

It turns out; this was a harder adjustment for me than it was for them. Once they became familiar with the routine and the foods, there wasn't too much of a fight to get them to do it. Me on the other hand, I've been living my unhealthy lifestyle for over 20yrs. It was my comfort zone. The food was good and exercising was hard. I had to find some kind of way to discipline myself.

One day, my mom came over and I was explaining to her that I was having the hardest time trying to eat vegetables. She suggested trying it as a smoothie. I would basically mix fruits and vegetables in a blender and drink it, instead of eating it. I was hesitant about the idea, but I felt like that would be more tolerable. She told me about a book she had called, 10-Day Smoothie Cleanse by J. J. Smith. This author put together smoothie recipes that were not only healthy but would cleanse your system. Along with the 10-day cleanse, she has various other smoothie recipes for various other reasons. She has meal prep ideas, so that you can eat healthy while drinking your smoothie. She even has smoothie recipes that are specifically for kids. I felt like this was just what I needed. I began to plan my 10 smoothie cleanse.

FEELING GOOD, FEELING GREAT

Change is hard at first, messy in the middle
And gorgeous at the end
—Robin Sharma

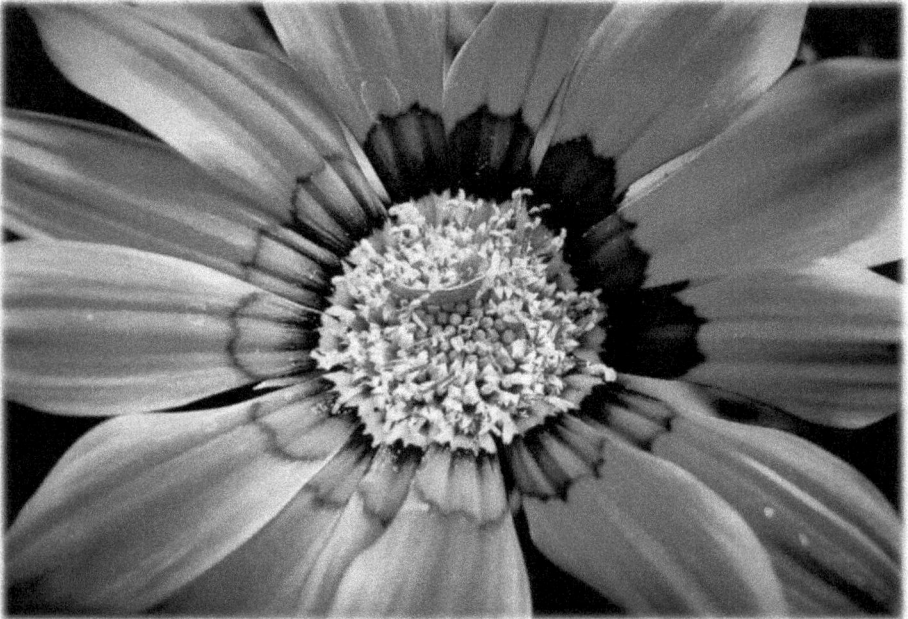

I must say, this lifestyle change was not all that bad. Of course it was a constant battle, but once you start seeing results, it pushes you even harder to stick with it. I started feeling amazing. Once I started to cut back on my unhealthy eating habits and added more fruit and water to the menu, I started feeling amazing. I wasn't as drowsy as I used to be. I had more energy to work out and chase my kids around. I didn't feel as stressed as I normally would.

I also noticed a change in my children. They started choosing playing outside over sitting in front of the game. They wanted to have their fruit and veggie parties for lunch. I didn't have such a hard time getting them up in the morning and getting them to bed at night. They were mastering the routine and the healthy foods without even realizing it.

I had my exercise routine down. I started drinking water after my work out, instead of juice. Even after my work out, I had so much energy. It was impossible for me to take a nap during the day anymore. I had to find activities to do to keep me occupied and moving. This was the best feeling in the world.

One thing I did to keep me moving, was walk. I would walk all around the neighborhood for hours, when my kids were gone. It was just something about nature and being outdoors that felt so good. That was my time to clear my head or think through my problems. I would have no set destination; I just started walking and went wherever my feet took me. I would usually walk in the evening. That way, by the time I got back home and showered, my body would be ready to rest for bed.

Walking is also good for the children. It doesn't have to be a very long walk. It could be just a walk around the neighborhood. It keeps them active and tires them out. This would be a good time to start learning how to run. When I would walk with my kids, they always wanted to race. So we would stop at a street lamp and race to the next one. It was hard for me at first. But as I continued to do it, it became much easier.

I've never felt that good in my life. It's amazing what change can do to a person.

THE SMOOTHIE CLEANSE

Your body is your temple. Keep it pure
And clean for the soul to reside in
—B.K.S. Iyengar

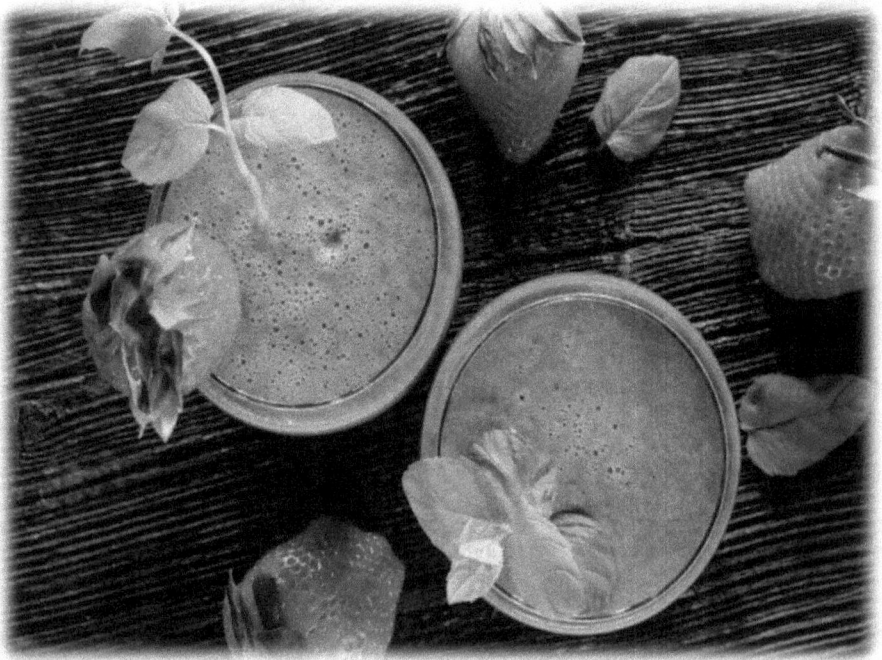

The day had finally come. I had all of the ingredients I needed to start my smoothie cleanse. The plan was to have nothing but smoothies for breakfast lunch and dinner for 10 days straight. I planned to drink one when I got up in the morning, the next one after my workout and the third one about an hour or two before bed. I finished all of my juice that I had in the house and didn't buy any junk food. That way I wouldn't be tempted to cheat. I wouldn't eat any solid foods. The only other thing I could have was water. Here is how my days went:

Day 1

This here is the moment of truth. I am making my first smoothie. Ever. I am so scared because I may not like it. But I am trying to hold onto hope since there is fruit included. Ok, here it goes.

Hmmm not too bad. I don't really taste the vegetables too much. I can taste the apples though. This isn't going to be too bad.

Day 2

So, today is not that much of a difference from yesterday. The flavor is a little different but nothing I can't handle. I am noticing that I am going to the bathroom a little more. Maybe this really is cleaning out my system.

One thing for sure, doing this smoothie cleanse and exercise together seems like a good fit. I think I can make it through this.

Day 3

I want food. I feel weak and my stomach is screaming at me. I need some food. I am trying so hard not to order me a pizza or take a trip to burger king. I want to eat. I couldn't even work out for a few minutes today. I don't know if I can do this. This smoothie is not enough for me.

Day 4

So, yesterday was horrible. I am feeling a little better only because I ate. I gave in and went to burger king. But, I also found a recipe in the book and made me a healthy meal. It was a chicken breast and a baked sweet potato. I made enough to last me a few days so that I wouldn't cheat again. Life is all about balance, right? So, I decided to do smoothies for breakfast and dinner and eat a meal for lunch. We will see how this works out.

Day 5

Today I am feeling much better than I have the past two days. The food really helped. I feel bad for cheating, but I can't lie, that burger was so good.

On another note, I was able to start exercising again. I am halfway there. I can't wait until this is over. Oh and today's smoothie is really good.

Day 6

Today, I noticed that my stomach had gotten a little flatter. I look thinner than I did before. I can't believe this is really working. I'm actually getting my fruits and veggies for the first time in my life and seeing results while doing it. I love this.

Ok, so its dinner time and I cheated. I had a slice of pizza. I felt like I needed to be rewarded for my hard work and I wanted it so bad. I will get back on track.

Day 7

I'm so over this cleanse. I didn't even finish it for today. I just want to eat food. I'm tired of this green stuff. And today's smoothie was not as good as the other ones. I am really going to try to stay strong. I really don't want to do this no more.

Day 8

I quit. There is no way I am drinking this smoothie today. It's so nasty. It's thick and lumpy. I just can't do it. I'm done.

Don't judge me. Yes I did quit. But I did well for it to be my first time. That cleanse just took me through so many emotions. Maybe there was a better way to do it, I don't know. But I decided I would take a break and maybe try to find another smoothie I can drink on a daily basis. I just needed to be able to eat food. I did my best stay away from pizza and burgers for the most part, after the cleanse. I just had to find what would work for me.

I did well for a while sticking to my routine. I decided to try out the weight loss smoothie. It was pretty good. This became how I got my servings of fruits and vegetables. I continued to use the recipes from the book for my meal plan. Don't get me wrong, I had cheat days. But over time I learned to discipline myself. I didn't have an urge to pick up sweets and juice when I went to the store. I even stopped going in the meat aisle, except to get some chicken breast. My body started to accept change and I was proud of myself.

I didn't completely give up on the smoothie cleanse. Since my mother did it often, I had help from her to try to get through the whole 10 days. If I messed up and stopped for any reason, I would just try again a few weeks later. It gets easier over time because you begin to know what to expect.

LET'S TALK RESULTS

Result happen overtime, not overnight. Work hard,
Stay consistent and be patient
—Gymaholic

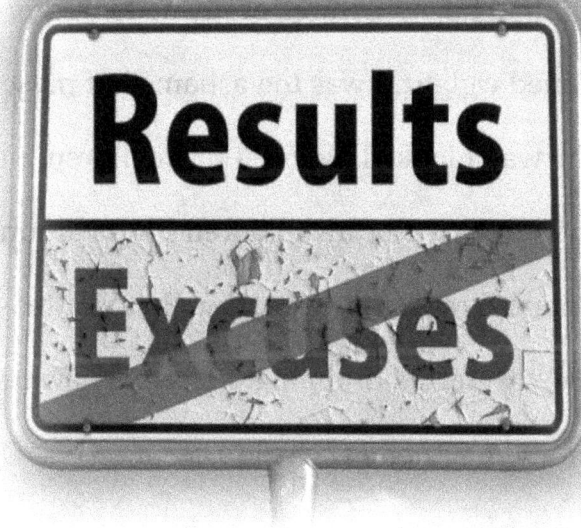

Now that you have an idea about some of the things I did to start my lifestyle change, let's talk about results.

It took me a while to see results because I would often fall off track. Sometimes things happened that were out of my control and needed my attention. There were times when the kids were sick and I had to tend to their needs. It was a very long and challenging process. But once I developed a steady schedule, the results started showing.

I wish I had taken pictures of my body during the time that I had gained weight. I was too ashamed of myself and didn't like the way I looked. Before I had children, my weight stayed around 120lbs. After my children it was around 160lbs. After a few months of finding a routine that worked for me, my weight slowly started dropping. Before I knew it, I was 10lbs smaller and I actually started to see it.

Although I may have been losing weight when I was just exercising, it didn't reflect on the scale because when exercising, you gain muscle. So don't be discouraged by the numbers on the scale. Another thing that helped show results was the smoothie cleanse. Although I didn't finish the whole 10 days, the results were there. My stomach was flatter, my face didn't look as fat and I was actually able to get a pair of old jean up over my hips. I never thought that I would see the day, but I kept those jeans for inspiration and I'm glad I did.

As I said before, this is a process. It's one that you have to constantly work at to reach your weight loss or nutrition goals. It has to become your lifestyle so that you won't completely fall off track again. You have to include it in your daily routine so that you can remain fit and healthy. You have to keep it in your children's routine so that they won't have to learn the hard way. You just have to keep at it.

TIPS FOR MOTHERS BALANCING WORK OR SCHOOL AND PARENTING

Balance is not something you find
It's something you create
—Jana Kingsford

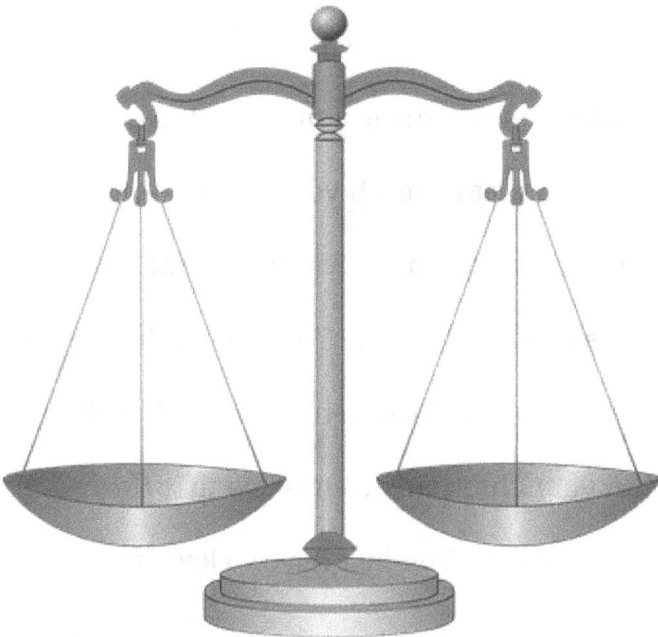

Of course I didn't forget about the working moms. I put my hands up to you all. Every now and then, I have to be a working mom and it is not at all easy. It's hard to find a routine for you and your children when you are gone half of the day. And for mothers that are in school, it feels nearly impossible, having to study and do homework. There are a few things you can do to fit fitness and nutrition in your busy schedule. Those things include:

Working moms

- If you have to be to work early, substitute that breakfast sandwich with fruit. It's healthy and it won't weigh you down.

- If you can, find a small workout routine you can do on your break or go for a little walk. It will give you a little more energy to get through your day

- If you can't exercise during your break, you can also try slipping into the gym after work or workout for 10min at night after the kids go to bed.

- Another great idea would be working out with your kids when you get home. They are going to want your attention anyway. So why not put some music on and dance

- Smoothies– I think they are great if you are on the go and for those 15min breaks at work. It's quick, easy and healthy.

- If you can't find time to incorporate exercise in your day to day life, get some friends together on your day off and go for a walk or to the gym. That way you will be exercising and having a social life at the same time

- Pack healthy lunches. Pinterest has a ton of meal prep ideas and snacks to include with your lunch

College Mom

- If you go to school on campus, you have a huge advantage. Every campus has a gym. If you have time between classes, bring some workout clothes and do a quick workout.

- Use the campus to your advantage. Do your homework or study in one of their quiet areas. This way when you get home, you can focus on your children and y'all routine. And you can squeeze in some exercise time. You'll have time to meal prep

- If you can't use the campus to your advantage, then remember routine. Come up with a schedule that accommodates your school work and your home. If you do this, your kids will learn it and they will know that during a certain time mommy is focusing on school work and when she's done she will focus on us.

- If all else fails. Ask for help. School can be stressful. Get someone to come to your house to keep the kids occupied so that you can take care of what you need to and decompress.

Whichever category you fall under, you can pick from the other category if it works for you. These are just some simple ideas to get you started.

MY THOUGHTS

The best preparation for tomorrow
Is doing your best today
—H. Jackson Brown Jr

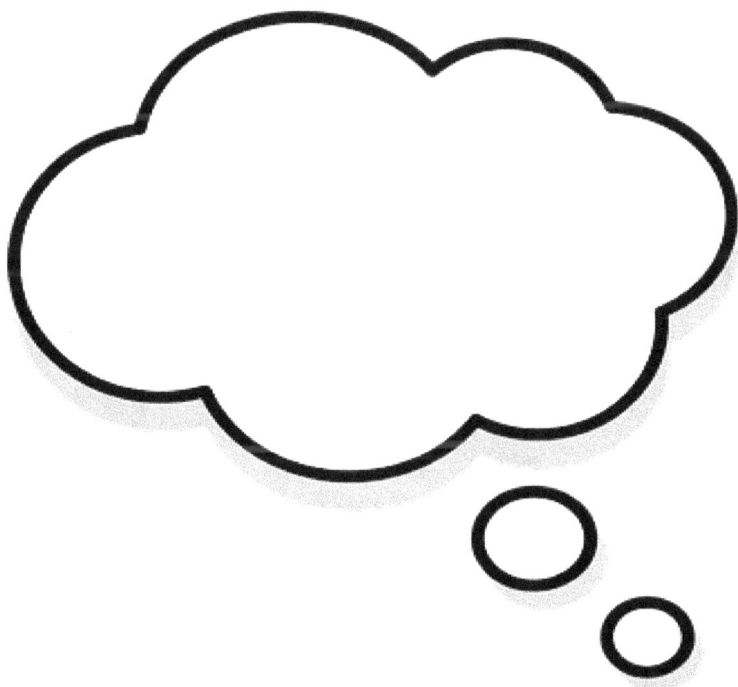

I am not a fitness expert by any means. I am not a nutritionist nor am I a life coach. I am simply a mother that wants to be around to watch her children grow into adults. It took years for me to get where I am. There were many trials and errors. But as I kept sticking to it, I found what worked for me and my family. Everything I've learned, I learned from research or family. There are so many free resources available to us to help us along our journey.

Don't wait until a doctor tells you that you have to change your lifestyle. You can start today.

What are you waiting for?

I created this section of the book to help you get started on your journey. You will find several different organizers to help keep track of things such as, your routines, weight and meal prep. I also included resources to find helpful healthy recipes for you and your children to enjoy. For an added bonus, I included my top 5 favorite YouTube channels. I wish you the best on your journey to a healthier life.

HOME ROUTINE PLANNER

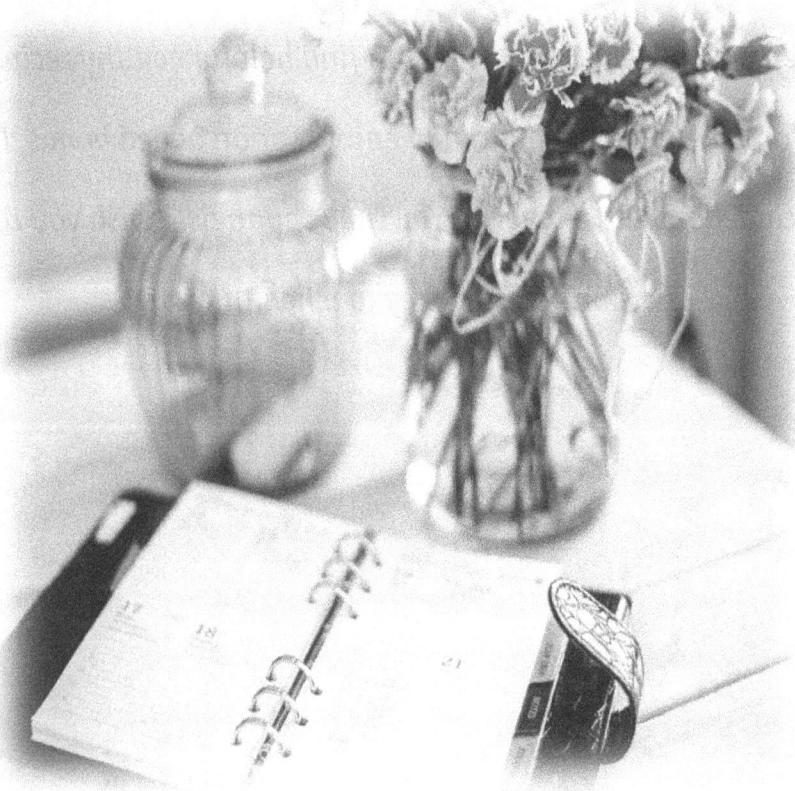

Morning

3am-_____

4am-_____

5am-_____

6am-_____

7am-_____

8am-_____

9am-_____

10am-_____

11am-_____

Noon

12pm-_____

1pm-_____

2pm-_____

3pm-_____

4pm-_____

5pm-_____

6pm-_____

Evening

7pm-_____

8pm-_____

9pm-_____

10pm-_____

11pm-_____

12am-_____

1am-_____

2am-_____

WORKOUT ROUTINE PLANNER

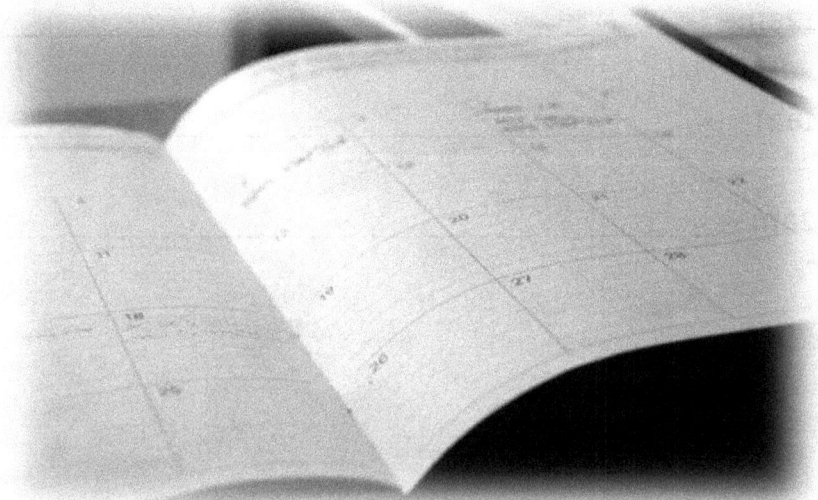

Days of the week	Exercise routine	Time Exercising
Monday		
Tuesday		
Wednesday		
Thursday		

Friday		
Saturday		
Sunday		

WEIGHT TRACKER

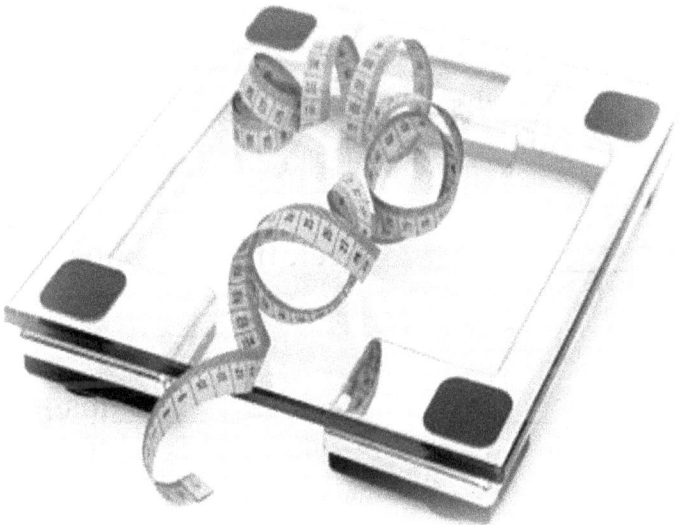

Start weight _____

Goal weight _____

Week 1 _____lbs   Week 7 _____lbs

Week 2 _____lbs   Week 8 _____lbs

Week 3 _____lbs   Week 9 _____lbs

Week 4 _____lbs   Week 10 _____lbs

Week 5 _____lbs   Week 11 _____lbs

Week 6 _____lbs   Week 12 _____lbs

GOAL TRACKER

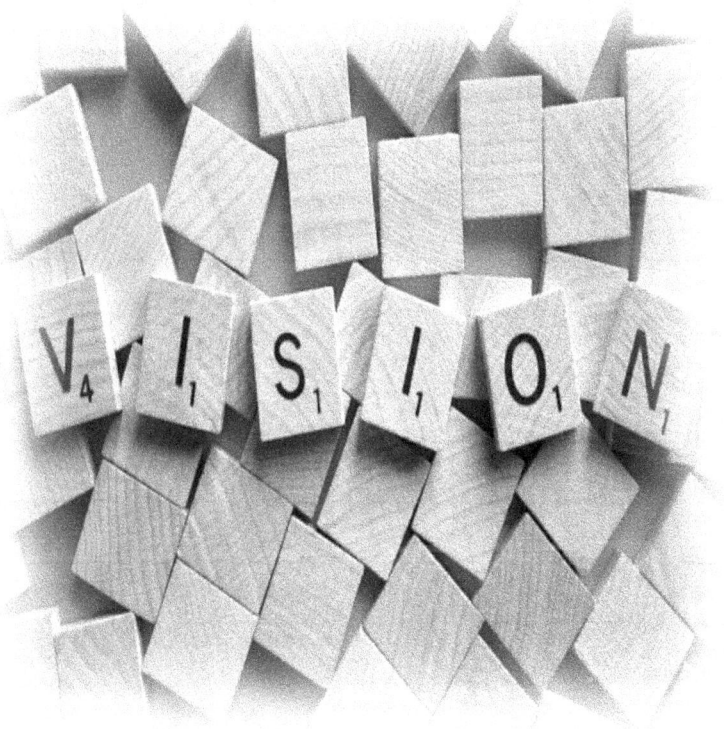

What are your fitness goals?

_____

_____

_____

_____

What are going to do different to accomplish these goals?

_____

_____

_____

_____

What areas on your body do you want to work on?

_____

_____

_____

_____

Find 5 YouTube videos that will help you with those areas.

_____

_____

_____

_____

_____

Which 2 videos do you see yourself keeping up with?

_____

_____

_____

_____

What are your nutritional goals?

_____

_____

_____

_____

What are you going to do different to accomplish these goals?

_____

_____

_____

_____

What about your eating habits need to change?

_____

_____

_____

_____

GROCERY LIST

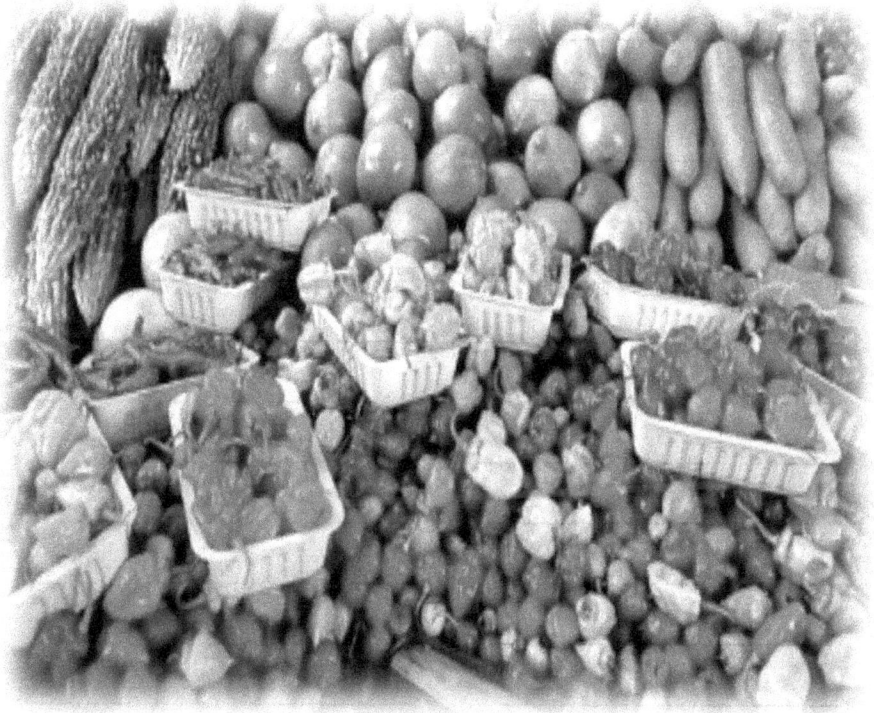

MEAL PREP TIPS

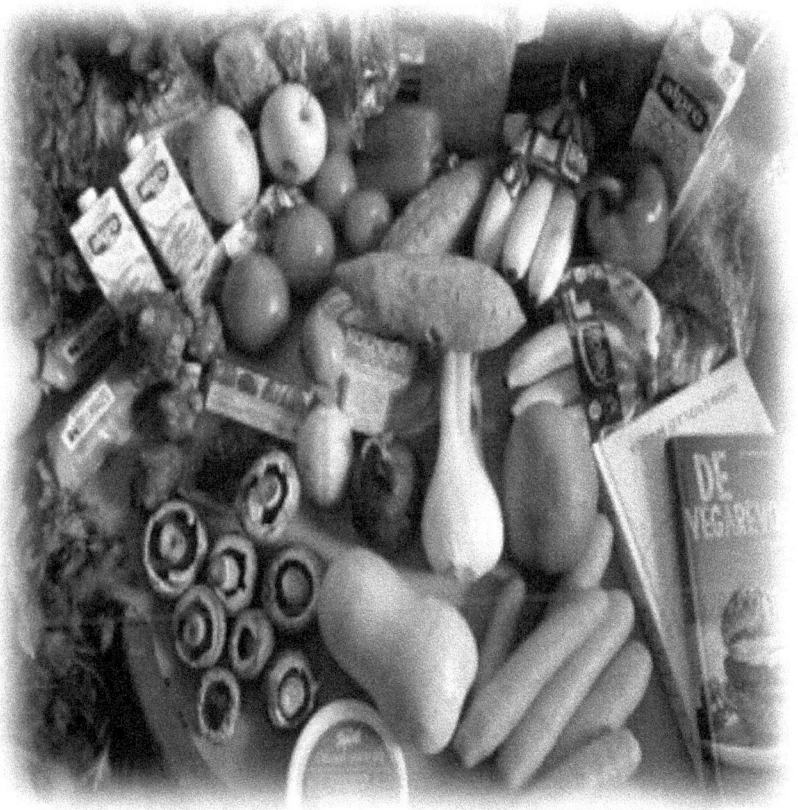

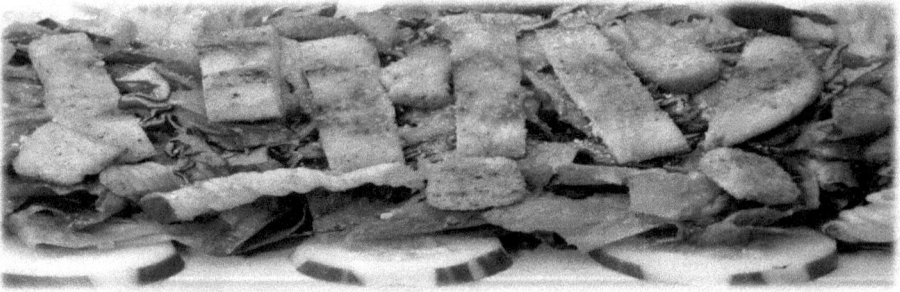

Below you will find some tips on things to consider before you start to meal prep. These tips can be found at http://skinnyms.com/meal-prep-beginners/. Check out their website, there is a ton of information on there.

1. Write down your goals– This helps you to decide which foods to eat and will keep you motivated during your journey
2. Choose a meal prep day– Schedule is key. Include this in your routine and you won's go wrong.
3. Decide which meals you're going to eat– Don't try to do it all at once. Do a few days' worth of meals or one day at a time if needed. Use freezer bags to separate the meals which will make cooking it faster and easier.

4. Choose recipes- This is important because if you choose the right food it won't be hard to stay on track. Do what works for you. Do what you know you like and add to it once you are comfortable doing so.

5. Get the right containers- There are tons of different containers. It is suggested that to make sure that they are BPA-free and that they are stackable for easy storage.

6. Make a shopping list- This will make the trip to the grocery store a lot easier. Figure out what and how much of each ingredient is needed and write it down. That way you know exactly what to look for.

7. Go grocery shopping- Stick to your grocery list. Don't pick up any unnecessary items. If you do have to get something, check the ingredients and make sure there are few ingredients listed and that you can pronounce them.

8. Prep- Get out your ingredients and start cooking

FITNESS/NUTRITION RESOURCES

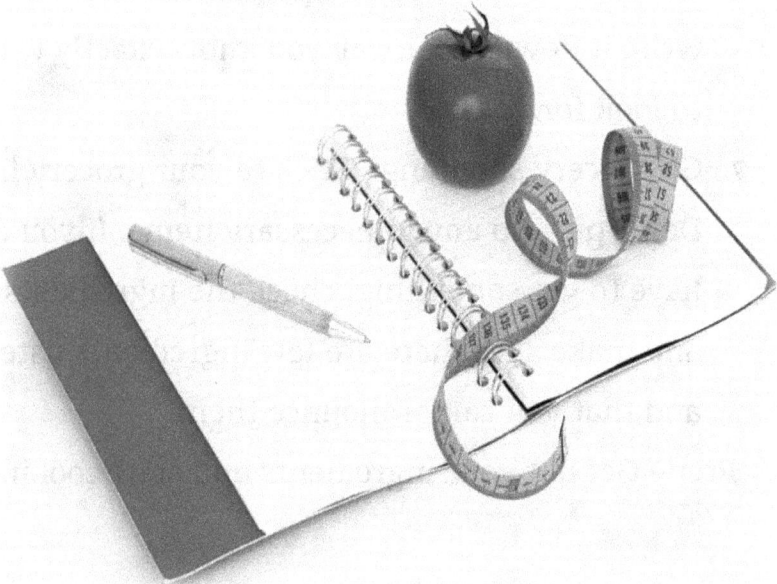

I found these websites on Pinterest.com

1. http://whatmomslove.comm – They have a delicious watermelon pizza that your kids are sure to love
2. www.inspirationformoms.com – Their backyard bug snacks are sure to be a hit
3. http://theimaginationtree.com – They have a list of 25 healthy snack ideas and 20 ice pop recipes for kids
4. www.dollarsprout.com – They give tips on how to meal prep spending under $50/week
5. https://healthyhappysmart.com -They provide you with a grocery list filled with healthy and clean eating choices
6. https://Healthylivingland.com – Gives great tips on how to teach your children to be healthy
7. https://simplelivingcountrygal.com – They give a step by step guide for beginner's meal prep
8. https://moneysavingmom.com – They show you how to prep 19 freezer meals in under an hour

I found these videos on YouTube

1. Brand It Britt – She is a transformation coach and she has an awesome personality. She focuses on fitness and nutrition. You can also find her on Instagram at KillerBodyNV. www.youtube.com/user/naturalvogue

2. Keaira Lashae- Along with exercise routines, she incorporates dance into her fitness. So you can learn dance moves while exercising. She can also be found on Instagram at KeairaLashae www.youtube.com/user/superherofitnesstv/featured

3. Remington James- His page is all about food but he does have great videos for beginner meal prep www.youtube.com/channel/UCO9Rhj_x_GgJI-Ria725EA

4. HealthNut Nutrition- Her channel is awesome. It's fun and colorful and filled

with a ton of healthy snacks, recipes and meal prep ideas.

5.   Whitney Simmons- Her channel comes with fitness exercises and tips for beginners. She also have nutritional videos on her channel www.youtube.com/channel.UCEQi1ZNJiw3YMRwni 0OLsTQ

6 DAYS	12 DAYS!	Black Women "Do" Workout! ABS-SO-TIGHTLY RIGHT! 24-Day Challenge	18 DAYS!!	24 DAYS!!!
5 crunches 5 leg raises 10 sec plank	20 crunches 20 leg raises 30 sec plank		75 crunches 40 leg raises 50 sec plank	120 crunches 50 leg raises 75 sec plank
8 crunches 8 leg raises 12 sec plank	Abs-So-Tightly Right! rest day		85 crunches 42 leg raises 55 sec plank	Abs-So-Tightly Right! rest day
10 crunches 10 leg raises 15 sec plank	30 crunches 30 leg raises 35 sec plank		90 crunches 42 leg raises 60 sec plank	130 crunches 52 leg raises 80 sec plank
Abs-So-Tightly Right! rest day	50 crunches 50 leg raises 38 sec plank		Abs-So-Tightly Right! rest day	140 crunches 55 leg raises 85 sec plank
12 crunches 12 leg raises 20 sec plank	65 crunches 33 leg raises 42 sec plank		100 crunches 45 leg raises 65 sec plank	150 crunches 58 leg raises 90 sec plank
15 crunches 15 leg raises 25 sec plank	Abs-So-Tightly Right! rest day		110 crunches 48 leg raises 70 sec plank	Abs-So-Tightly Right! rest day

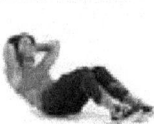

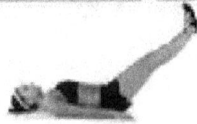

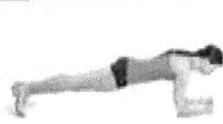

30 DAY EASY SQUAT
CHALLENGE
www.30dayfitnesschallenges.com

DAY 1	30 SQUATS		DAY 16	80 SQUATS
DAY 2	50 SQUATS		DAY 17	50 SQUATS
DAY 3	75 SQUATS		DAY 18	125 SQUATS
DAY 4	60 SQUATS		DAY 19	50 SQUATS
DAY 5	REST DAY		DAY 20	REST DAY
DAY 6	60 SQUATS		DAY 21	145 SQUATS
DAY 7	90 SQUATS		DAY 22	80 SQUATS
DAY 8	50 SQUATS		DAY 23	40 SQUATS
DAY 9	45 SQUATS		DAY 24	100 SQUATS
DAY 10	REST DAY		DAY 25	REST DAY
DAY 11	120 SQUATS		DAY 26	75 SQUATS
DAY 12	40 SQUATS		DAY 27	50 SQUATS
DAY 13	75 SQUATS		DAY 28	150 SQUATS
DAY 14	125 SQUATS		DAY 29	95 SQUATS
DAY 15	REST DAY		DAY 30	175 SQUATS

#30dayfitness   www.30dayfitnesschallenges.com   #30dayfitness

Shantel McCoy

Printed in the United States of America

ISBN- 978-1-7320662-1-2

www.ingramcontent.com/pod-product-compliance
Lightning Source LLC
Chambersburg PA
CBHW050547280326
41933CB00011B/1757